Care for
Mama Bear

was written in the hopes that it would be a helpful tool for parents, counselors, teachers, and anyone else who works with children. The goal of this book is to capture the essential, underlying concerns and fears some children have and can not articulate when coping with a parent or loved one that has cancer. It is a helpful reminder to children, that they will always be loved, and that they are not alone.

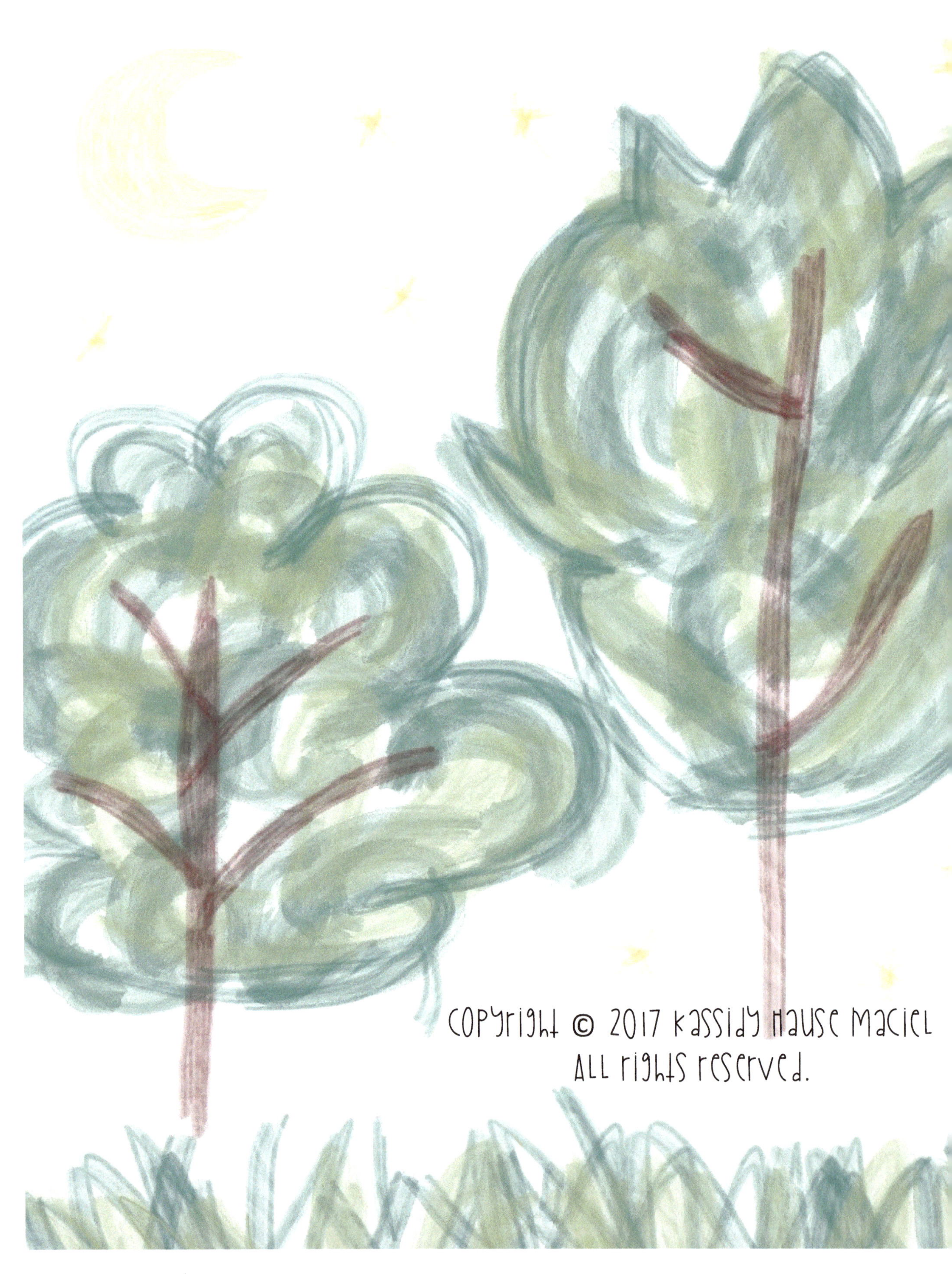

copyright © 2017 kassidy hause maciel
all rights reserved.

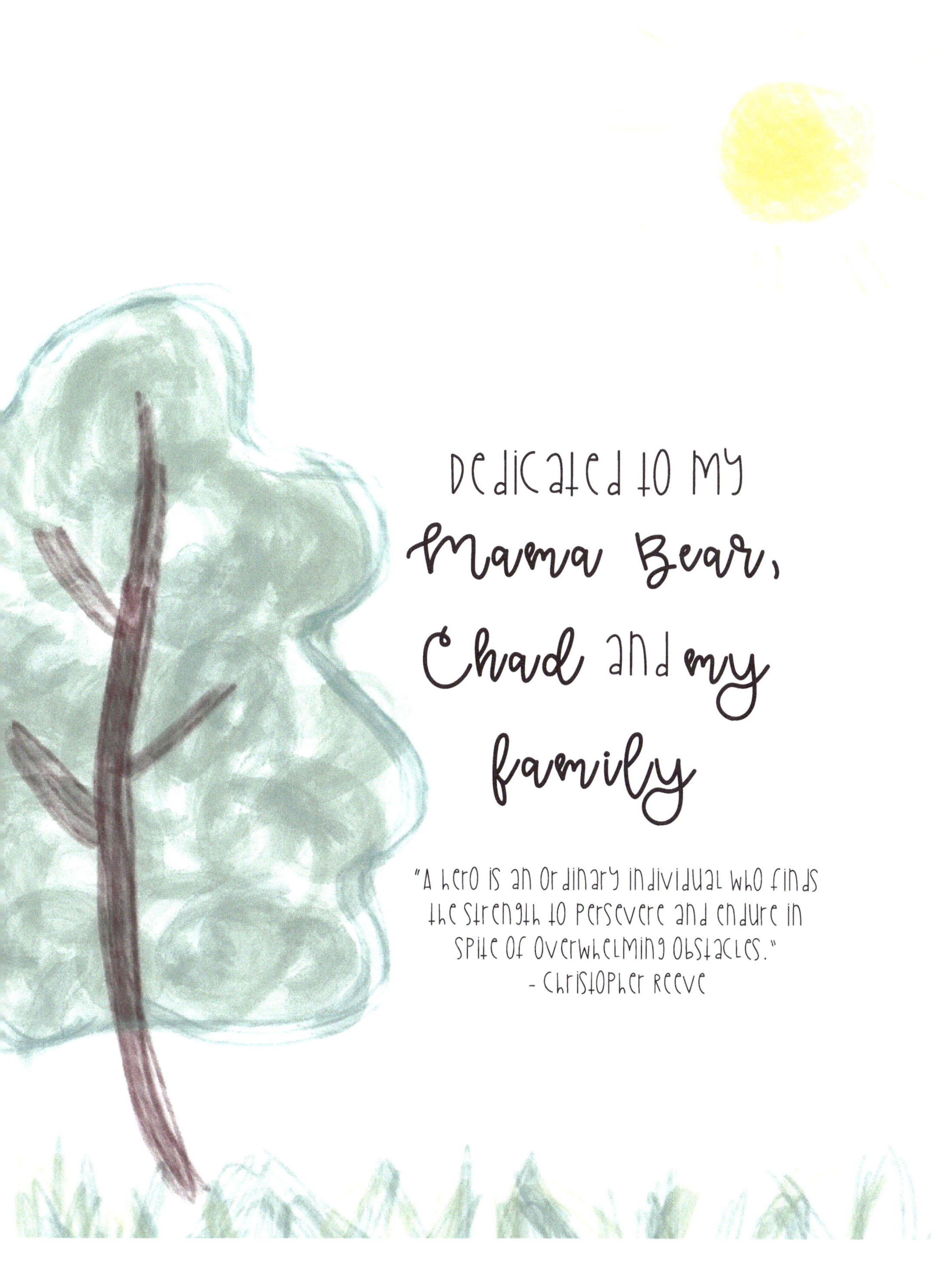

Dedicated to my
Mama Bear,
Chad and my
family
"A hero is an ordinary individual who finds
the strength to persevere and endure in
spite of overwhelming obstacles."
- Christopher Reeve

Hi there! My name is Marley.

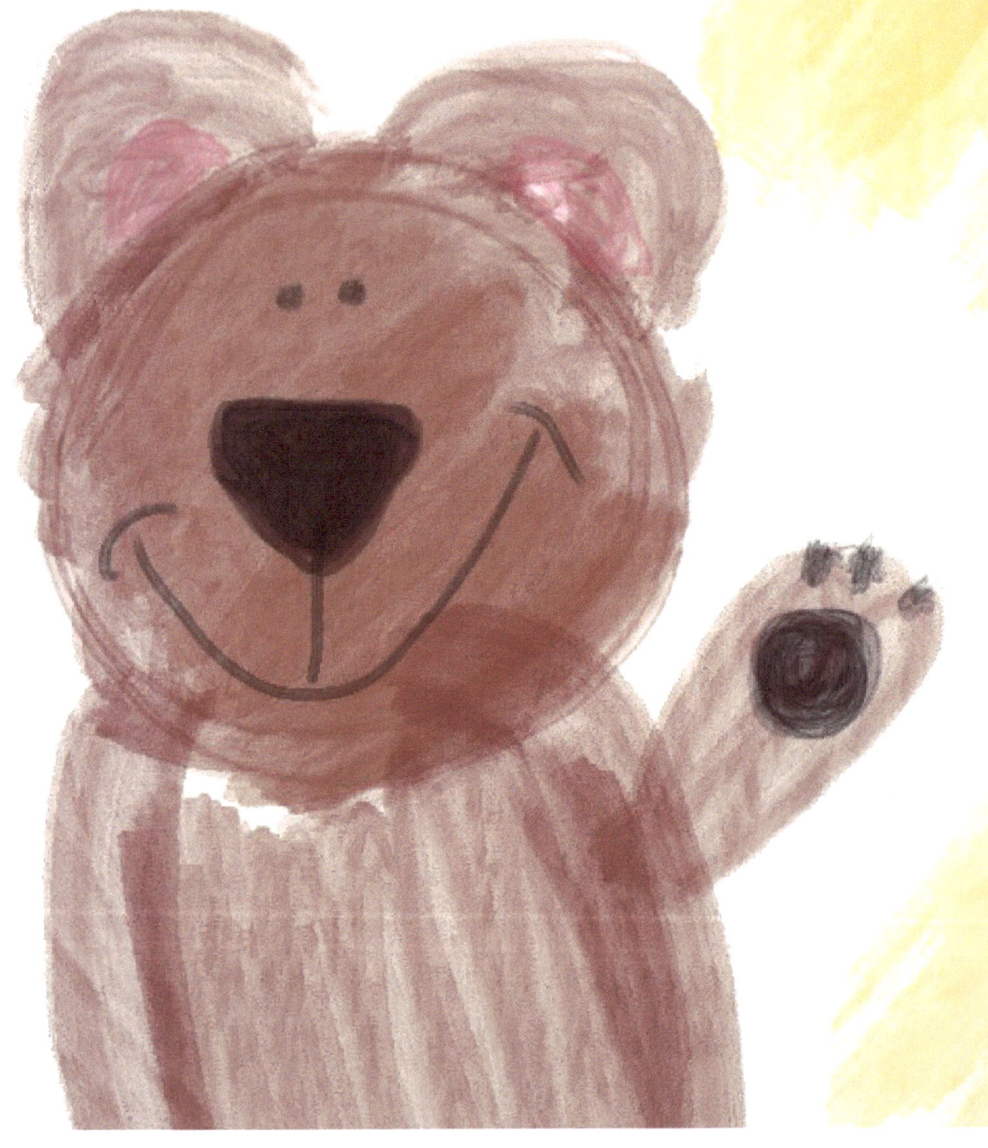

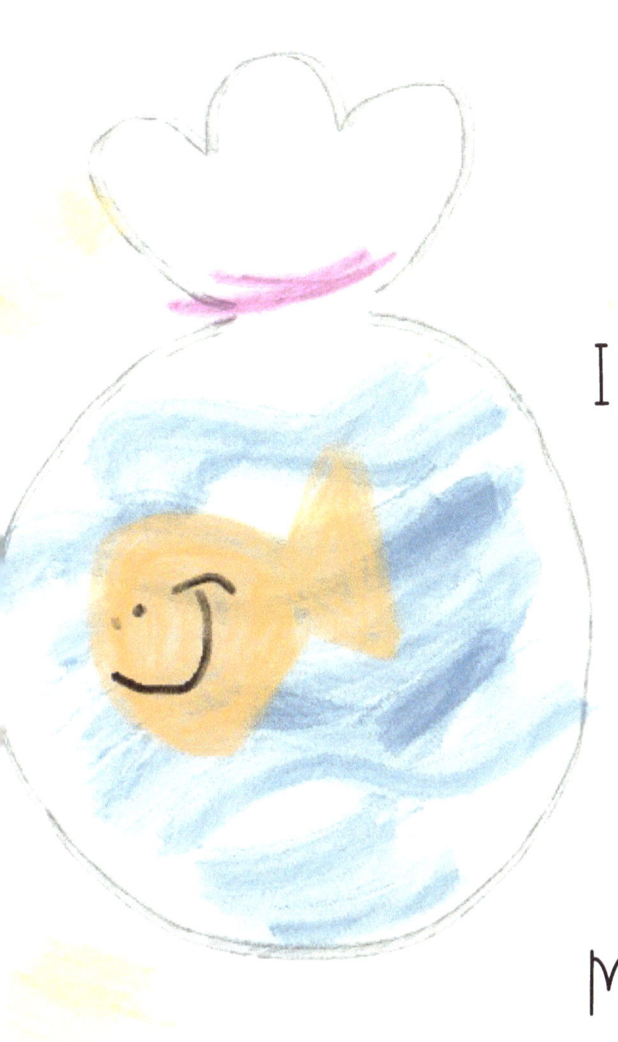

I am five years old.
I have a pet fish
and I love to play
soccer.

My life seems pretty
normal. In most
ways it is.
Except...

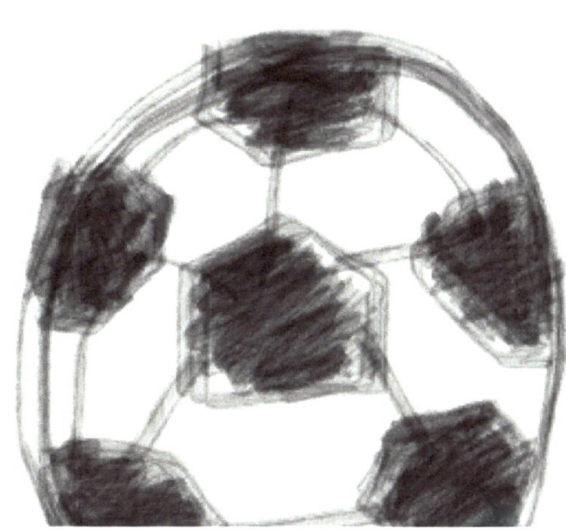

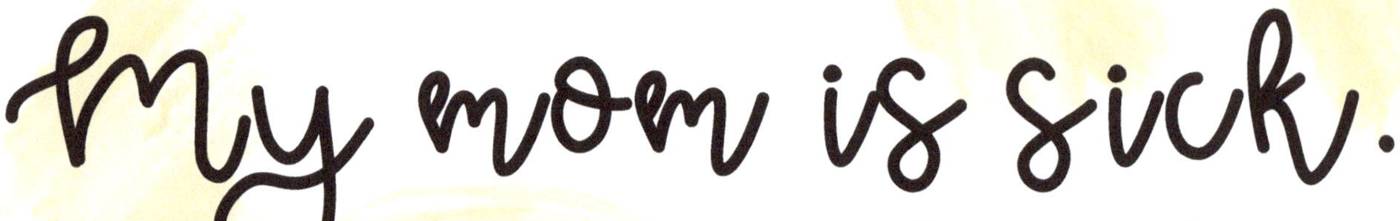

My mom is sick. 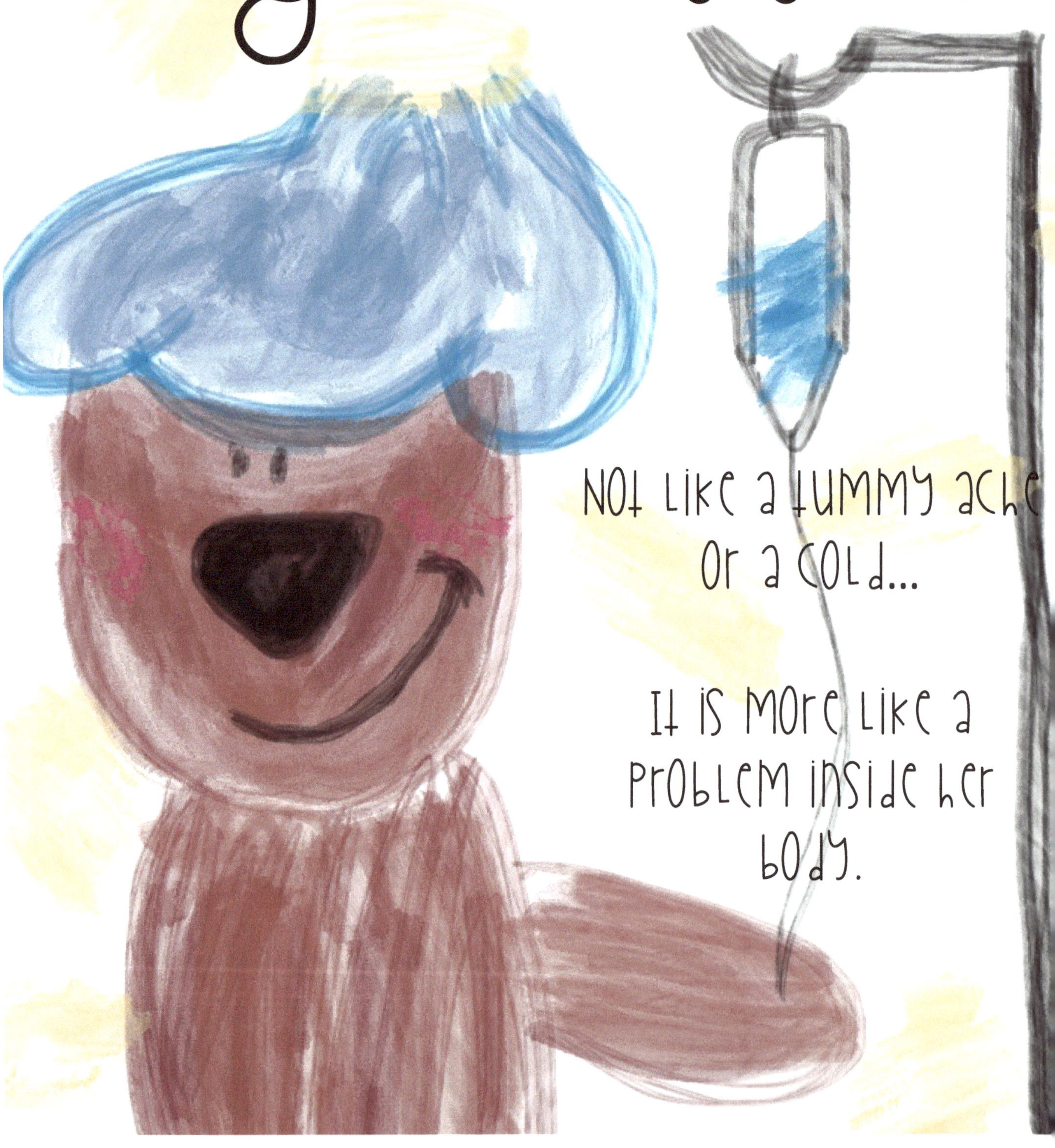
NOt like a tummy ache
Or a cold...

It is more like a
problem inside her
body.

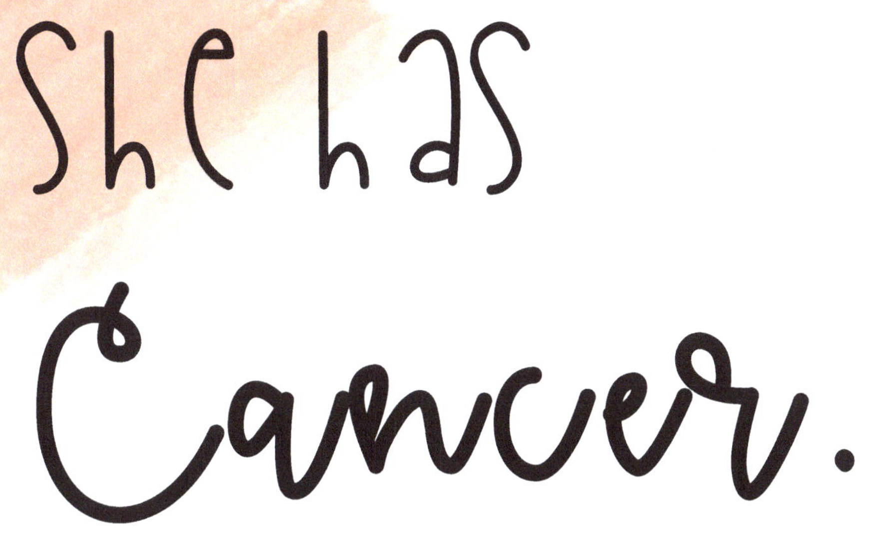
She has
Cancer.

I really wanted to know what cancer was and how I could fix it. So I asked my mama bear, "What is cancer?"

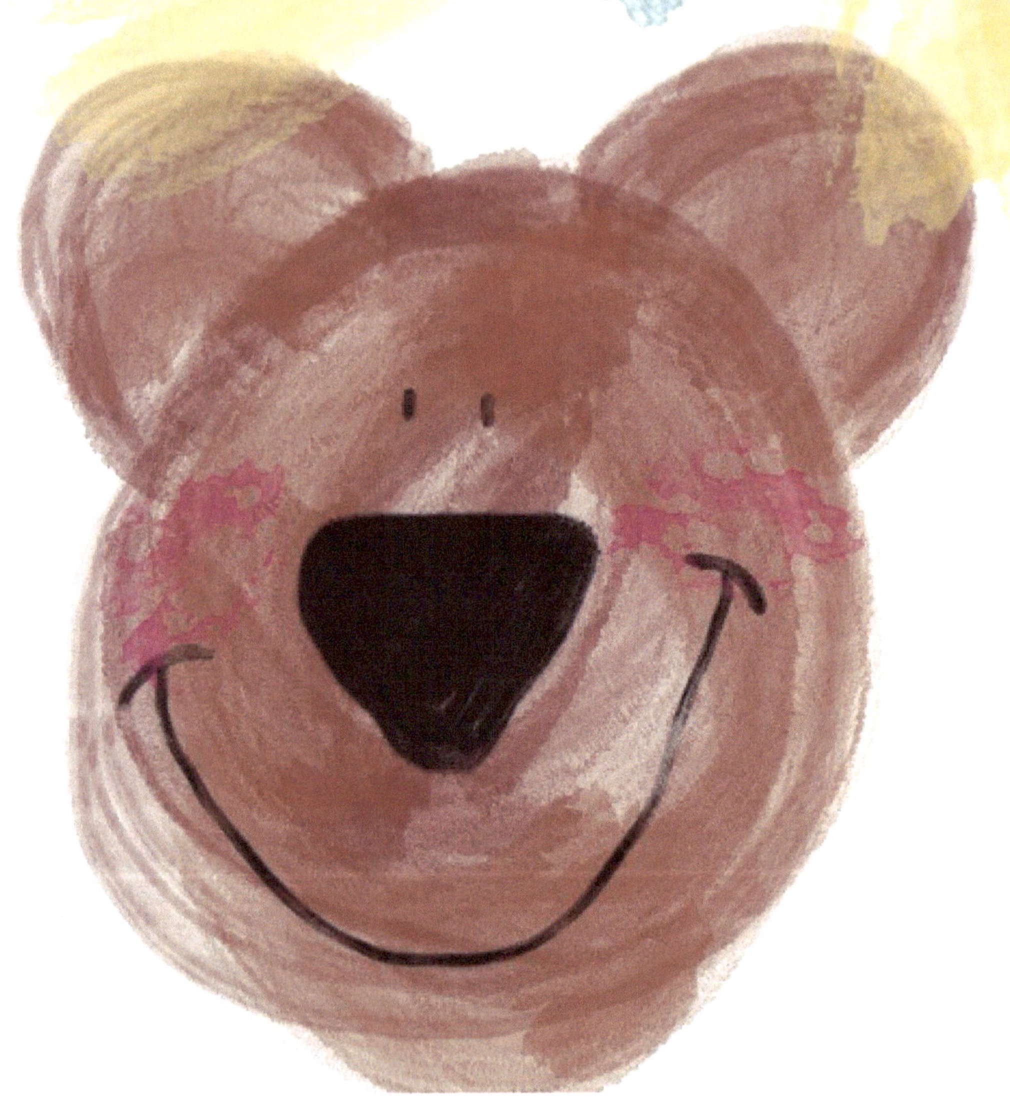

Cancer can be a scary word.
It is okay to feel scared,
worried, or
confused. I used to be
scared too, but talking to
grown ups about my feelings
really helped me feel
better.

She told me cancer is a type of sickness. It's when something is wrong with the inside of the body.

She told me that our bodies are made up of cells and cancer creates a lot of bad cells. The bad cells can also create lumps inside the body. That is why this sickness can last a long time.

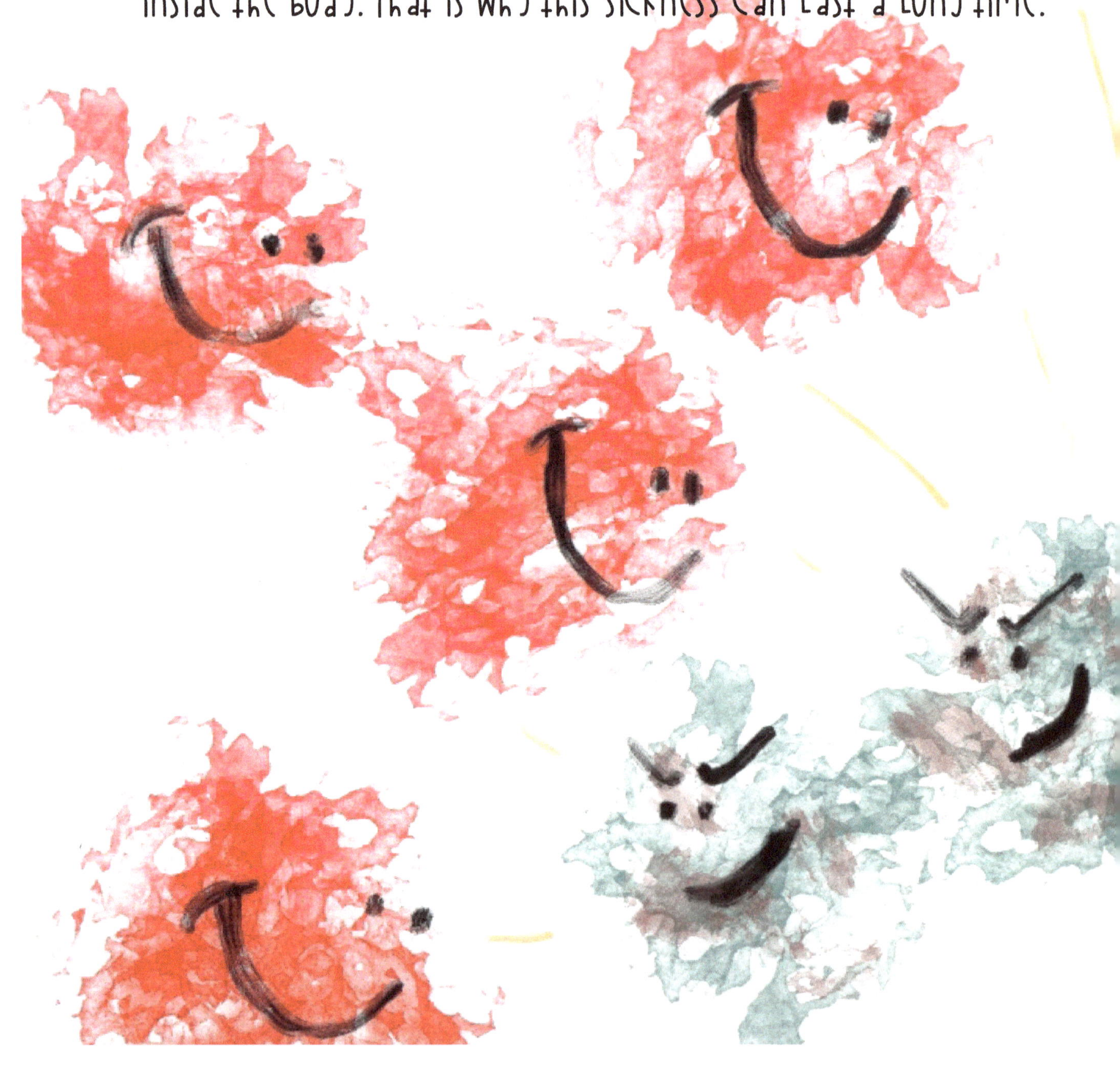

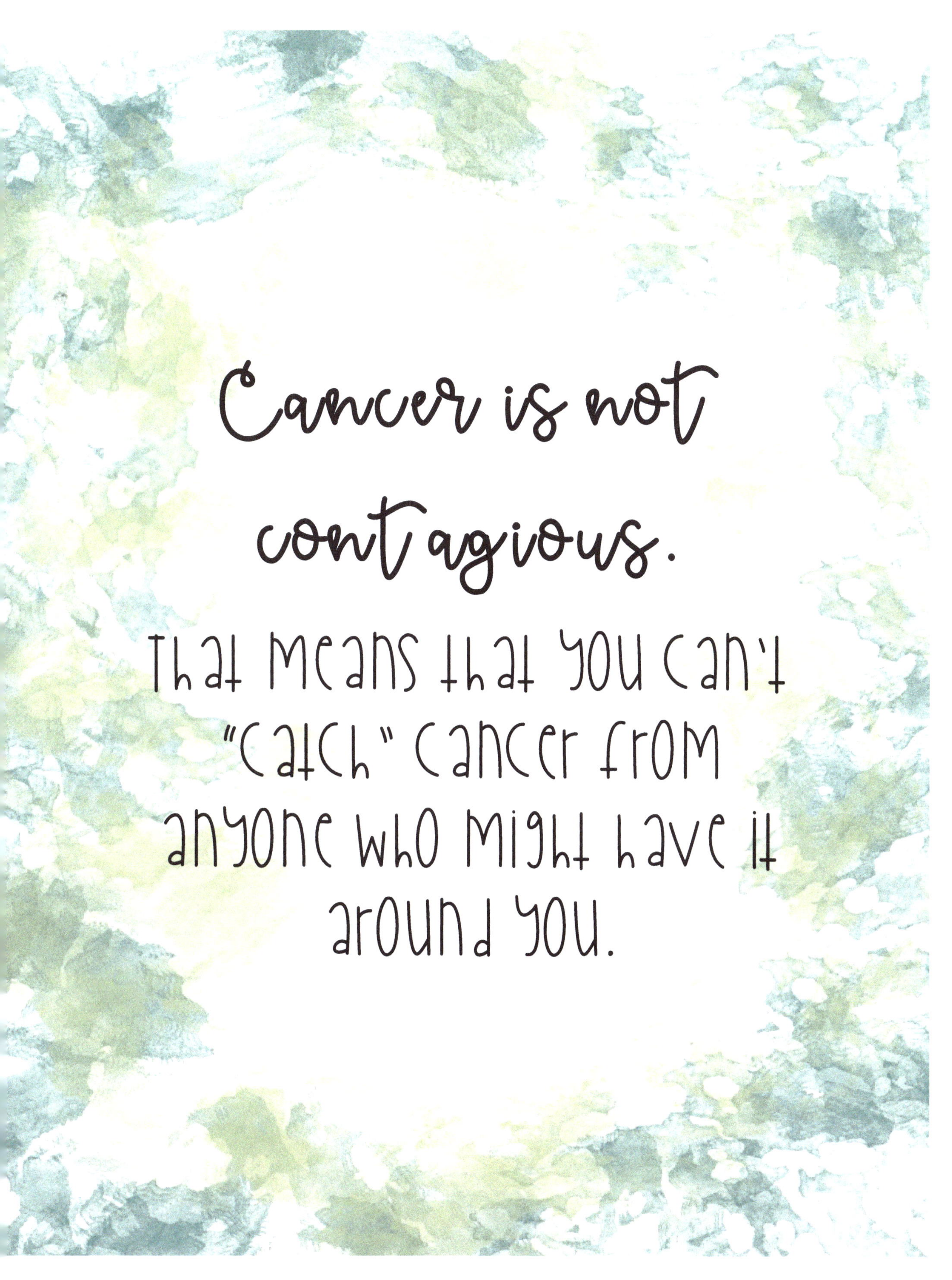

Cancer is not contagious.
That means that you can't "catch" cancer from anyone who might have it around you.

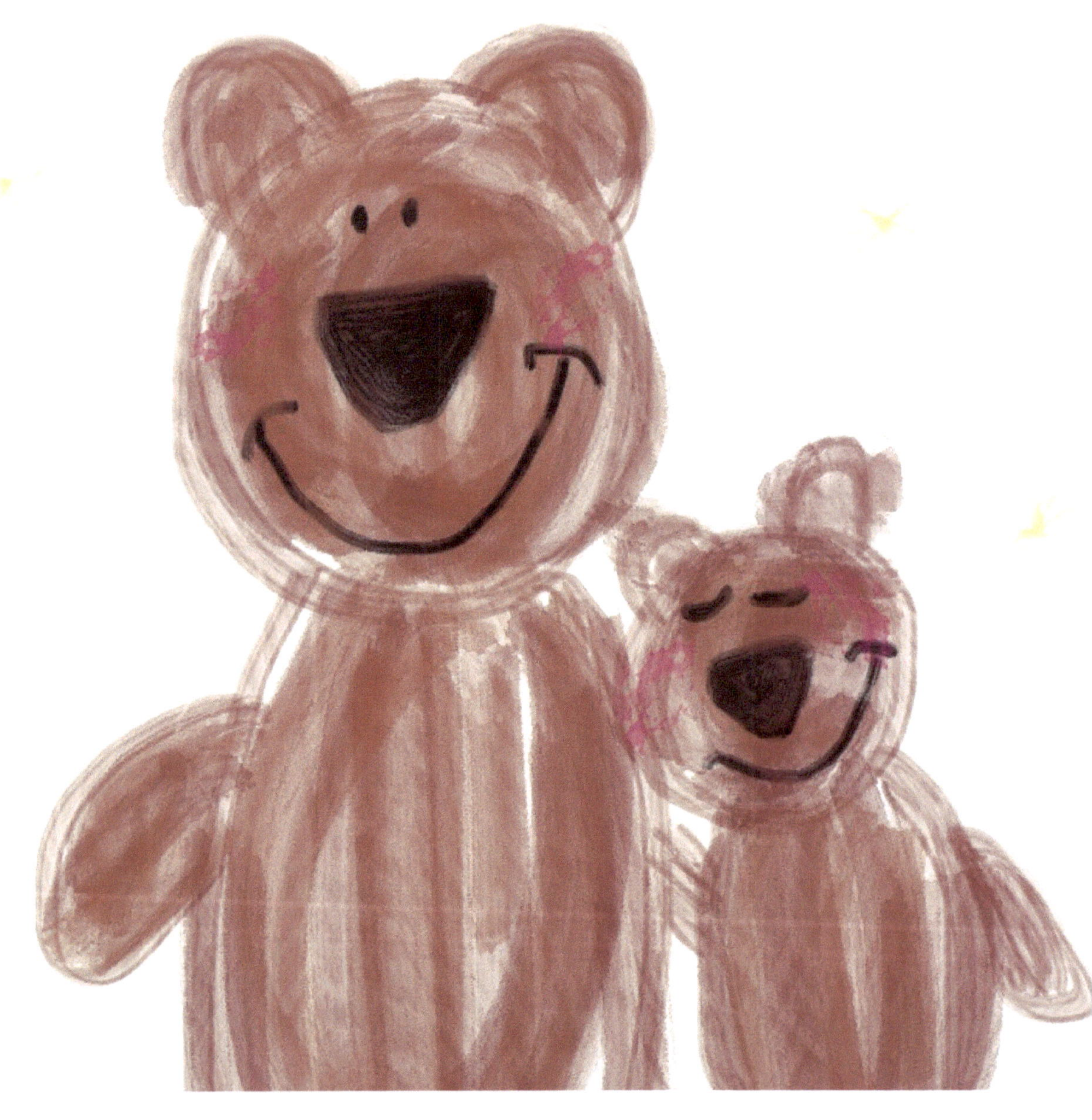

That means I can hug and kiss my
mom as much as I want.
(just between you and i, I am pretty
sure it helps her feel better).

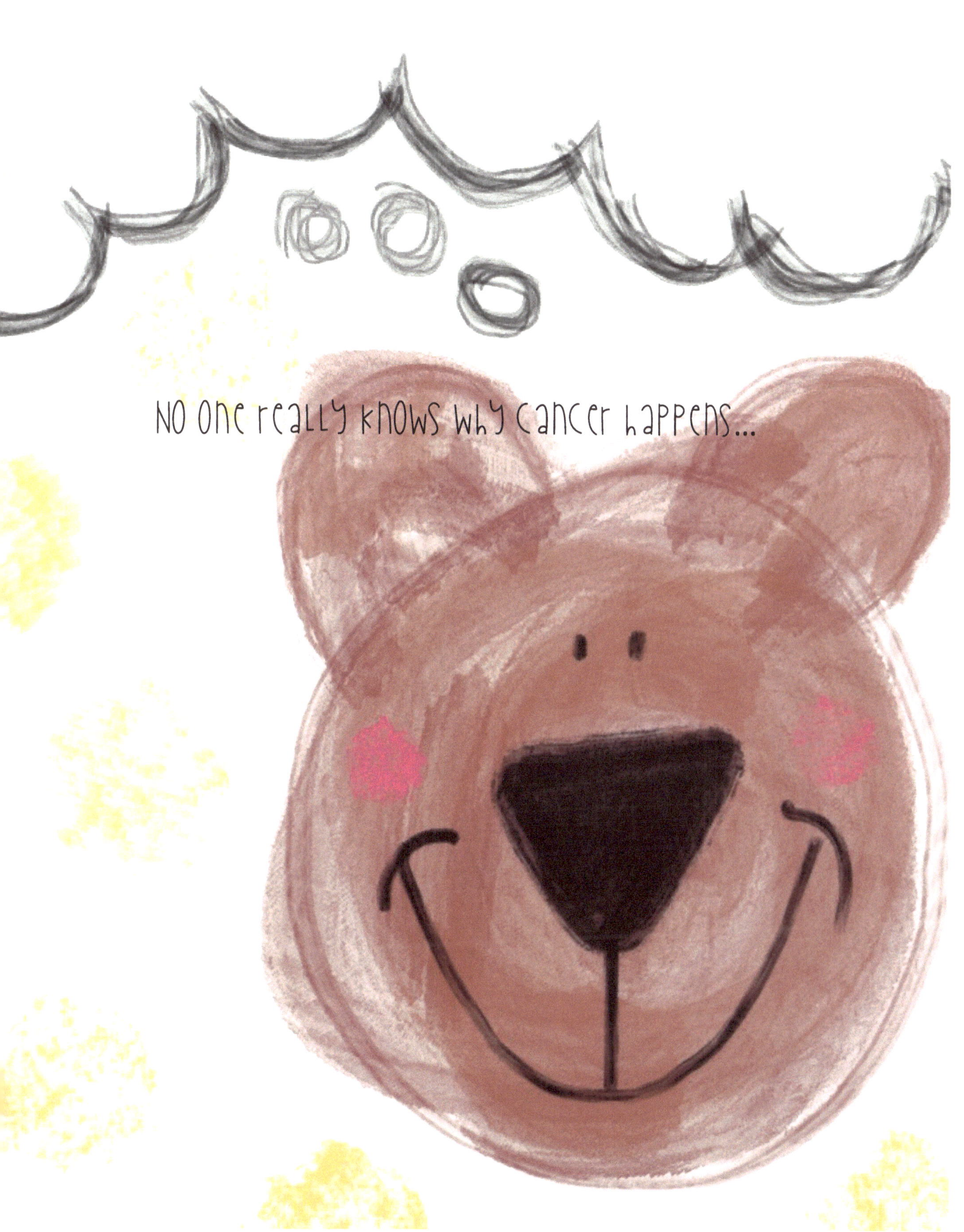
No one really knows why cancer happens...

But I do know that it is nobody's fault and no one can cause it.

Cancer just happens sometimes on its own and the only way to fix it is to go to the doctor and get the right medicine.

Here are just a few
things that **changed**

in my life when my
mom got sick...

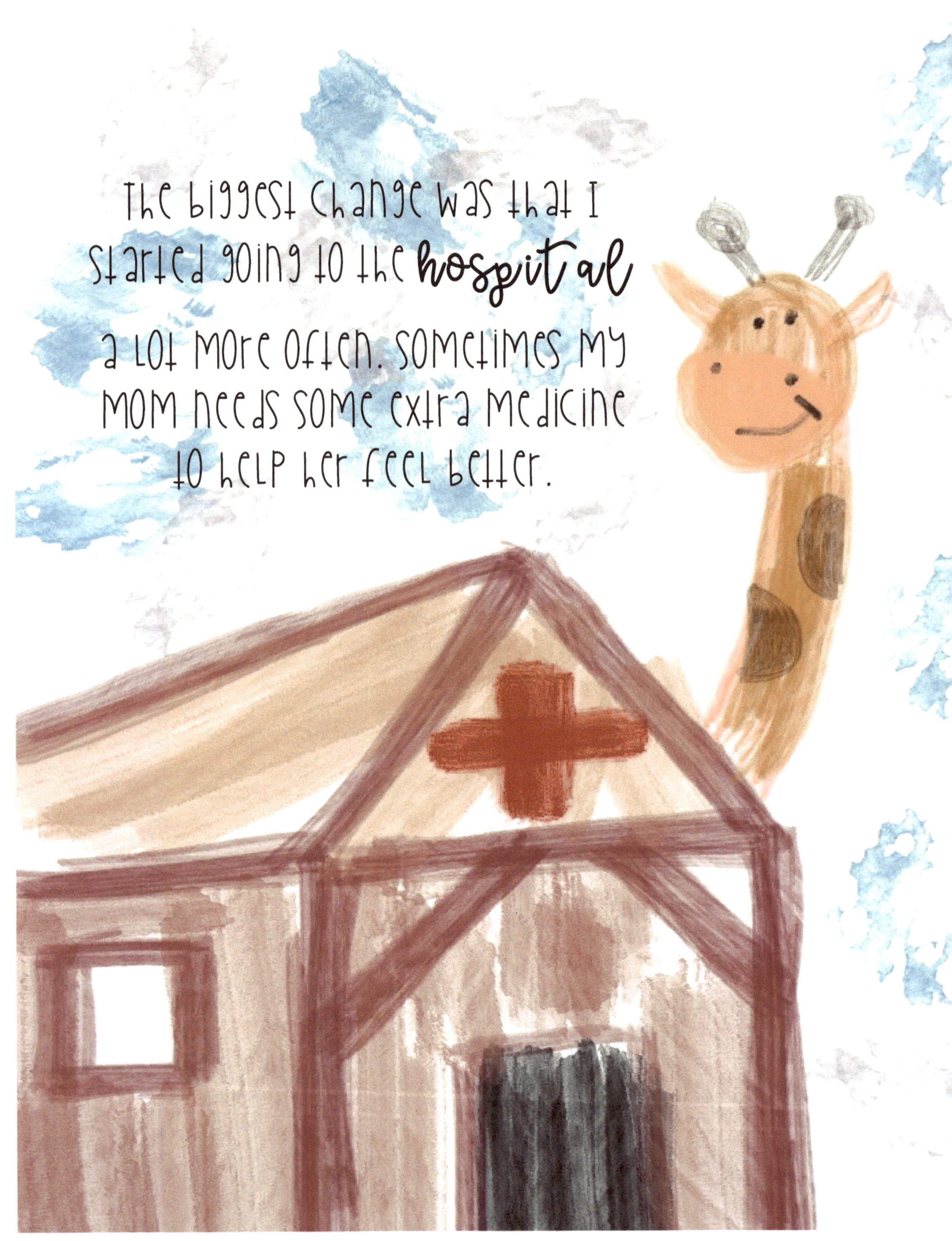
The biggest change was that I started going to the **hospital** a lot more often. Sometimes my mom needs some extra medicine to help her feel better.

Sometimes my family and I are at the hospital all day. I used to be scared I was going to have to live there! But that was silly of me. That would never happen!

We always come home when my mama is done getting all of her medicine to help her feel better.

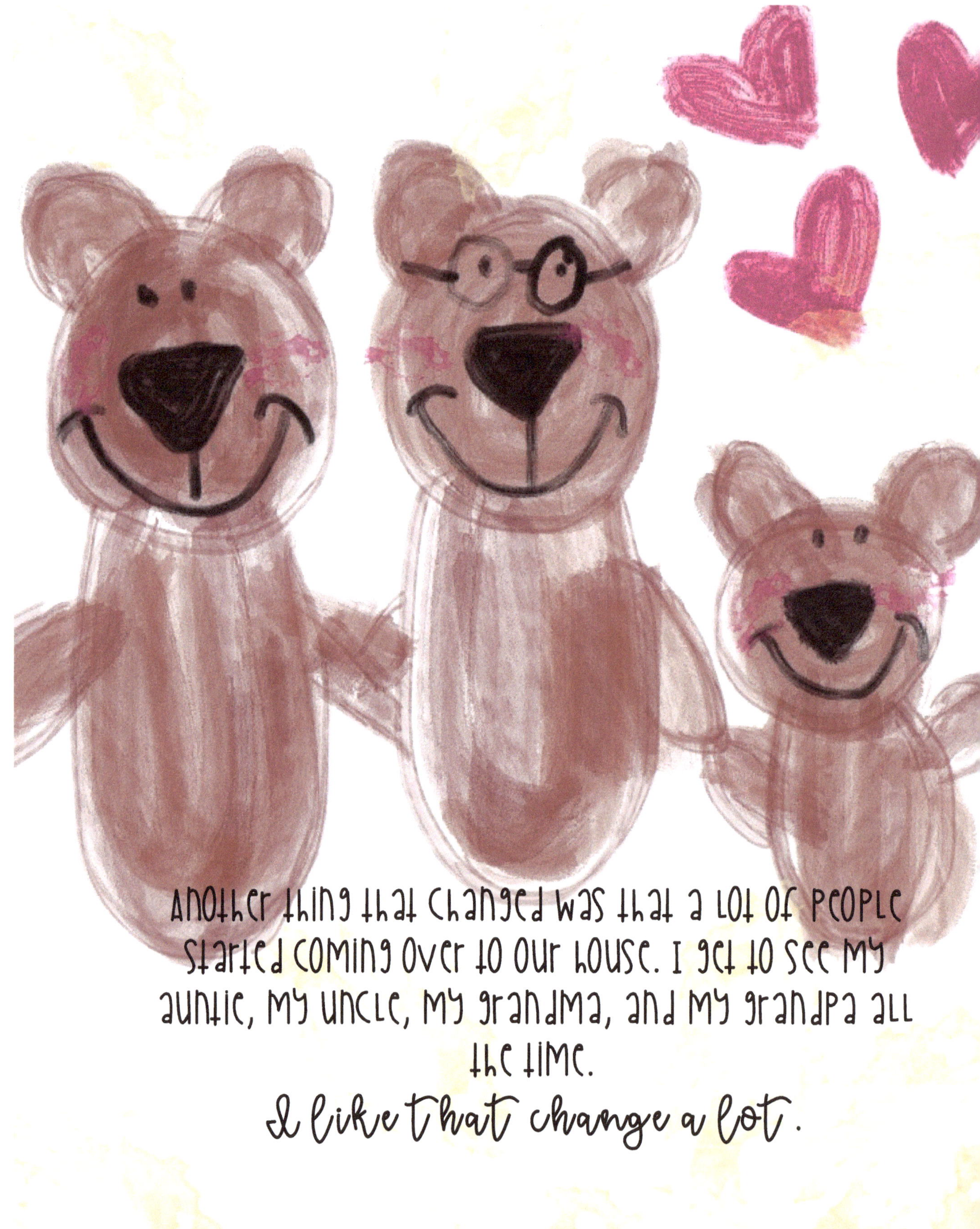

Another thing that changed was that a lot of people started coming over to our house. I get to see my auntie, my uncle, my grandma, and my grandpa all the time.
I like that change a lot.

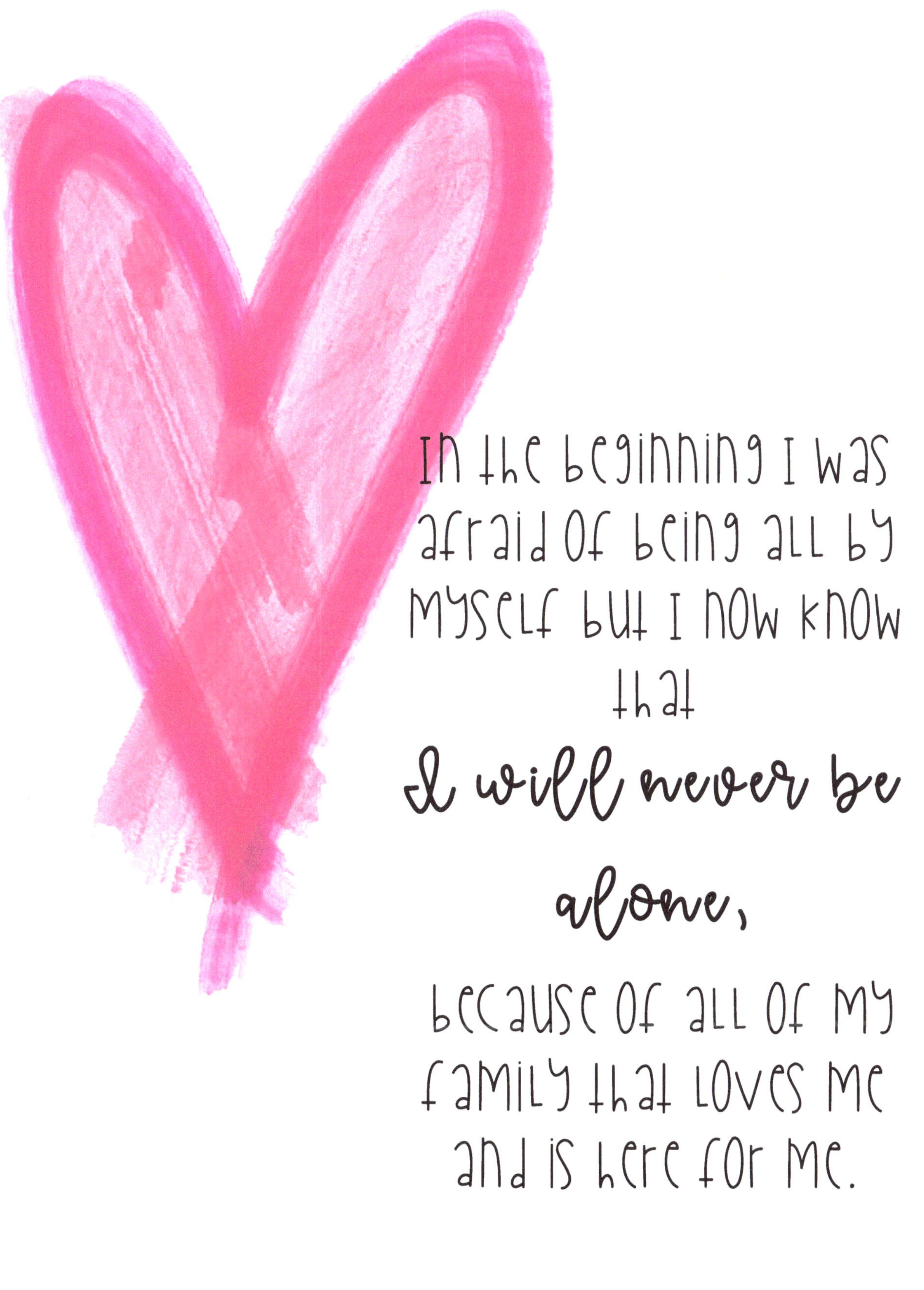

In the beginning I was afraid of being all by myself but I now know that
I will never be alone,
because of all of my family that loves me and is here for me.

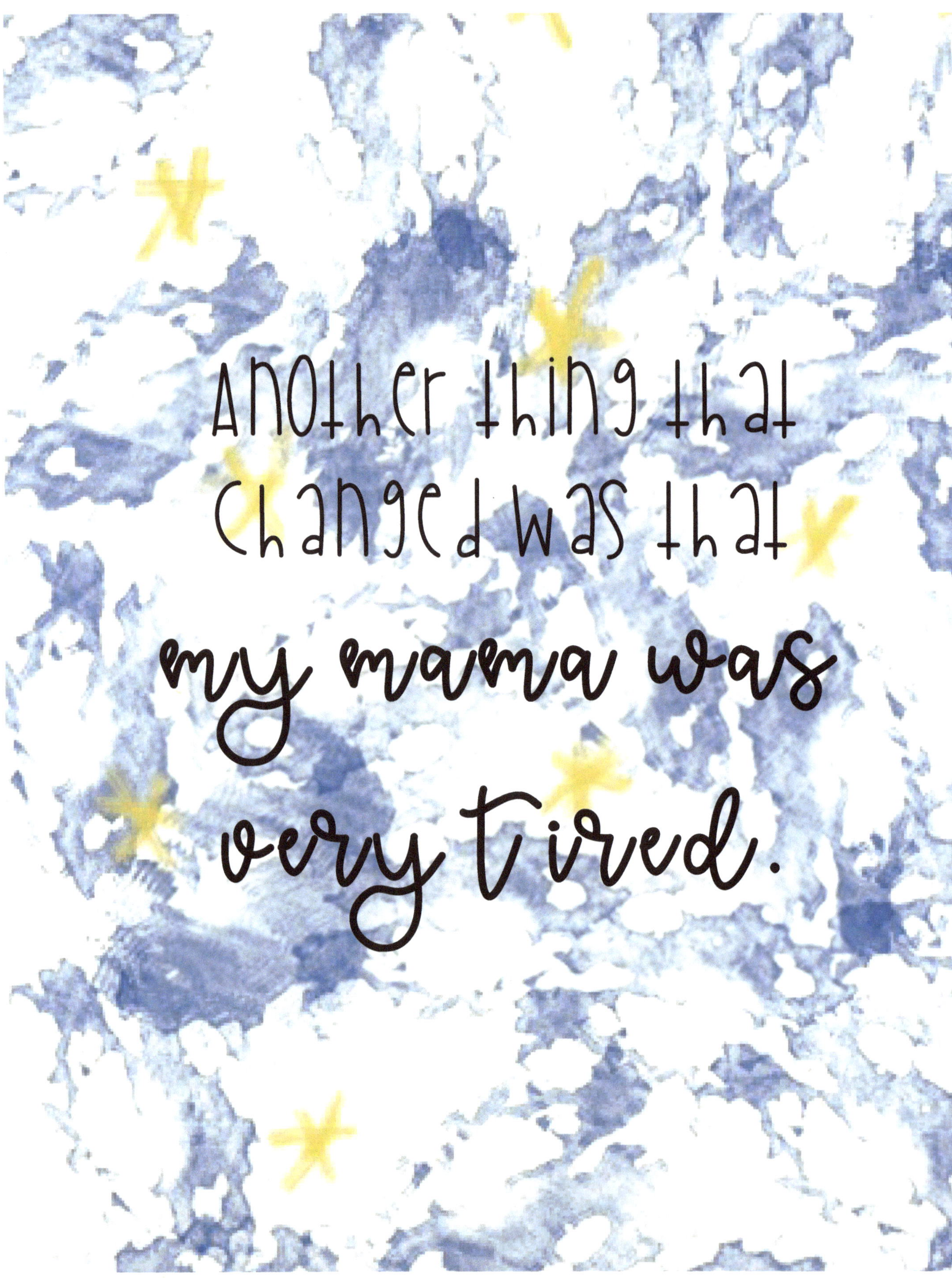

another thing that
changed was that
my mama was
very tired.

She told me that she gets very tired from her medicine she has to take but that she has to take it in order to make herself feel better. I want my mom to feel better so sometimes when she is too tired to play I will cuddle her in bed and we snuggle, eat popcorn, and watch movies.

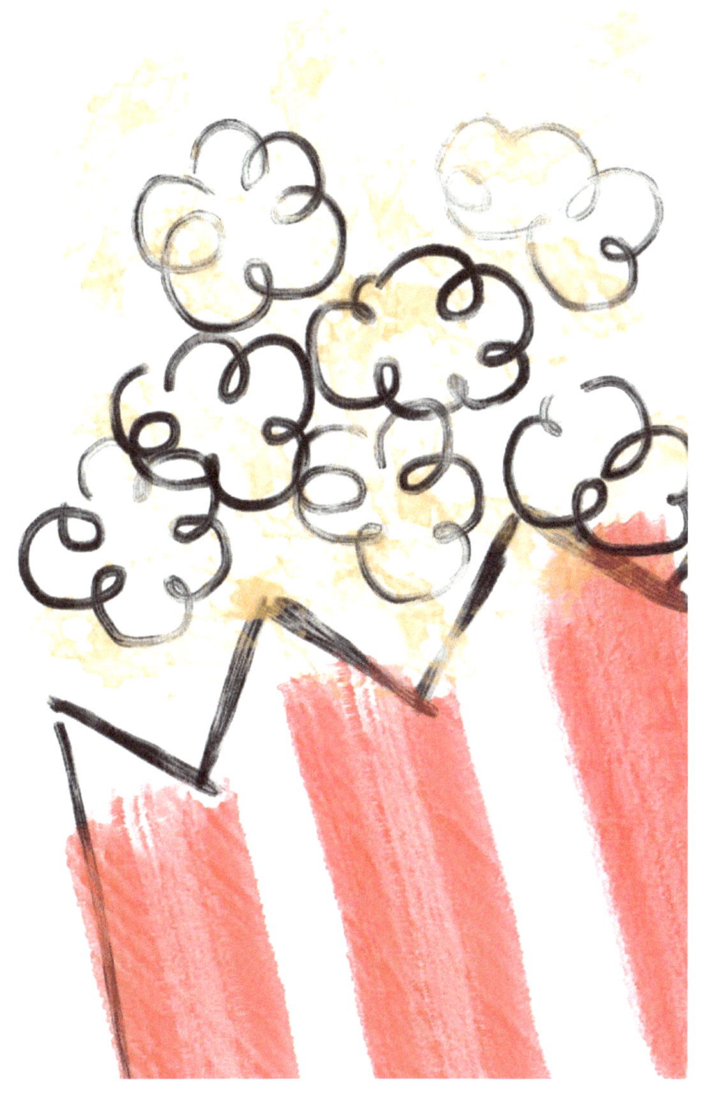

My mom also looks a little different too. She lost a lot of her hair and when I asked why she said it was because of the cancer medicine and that it is completely normal. She told me it would grow right back when she is done taking the medicine.

Even though she might look a little different on the outside she is still my same, beautiful mama.

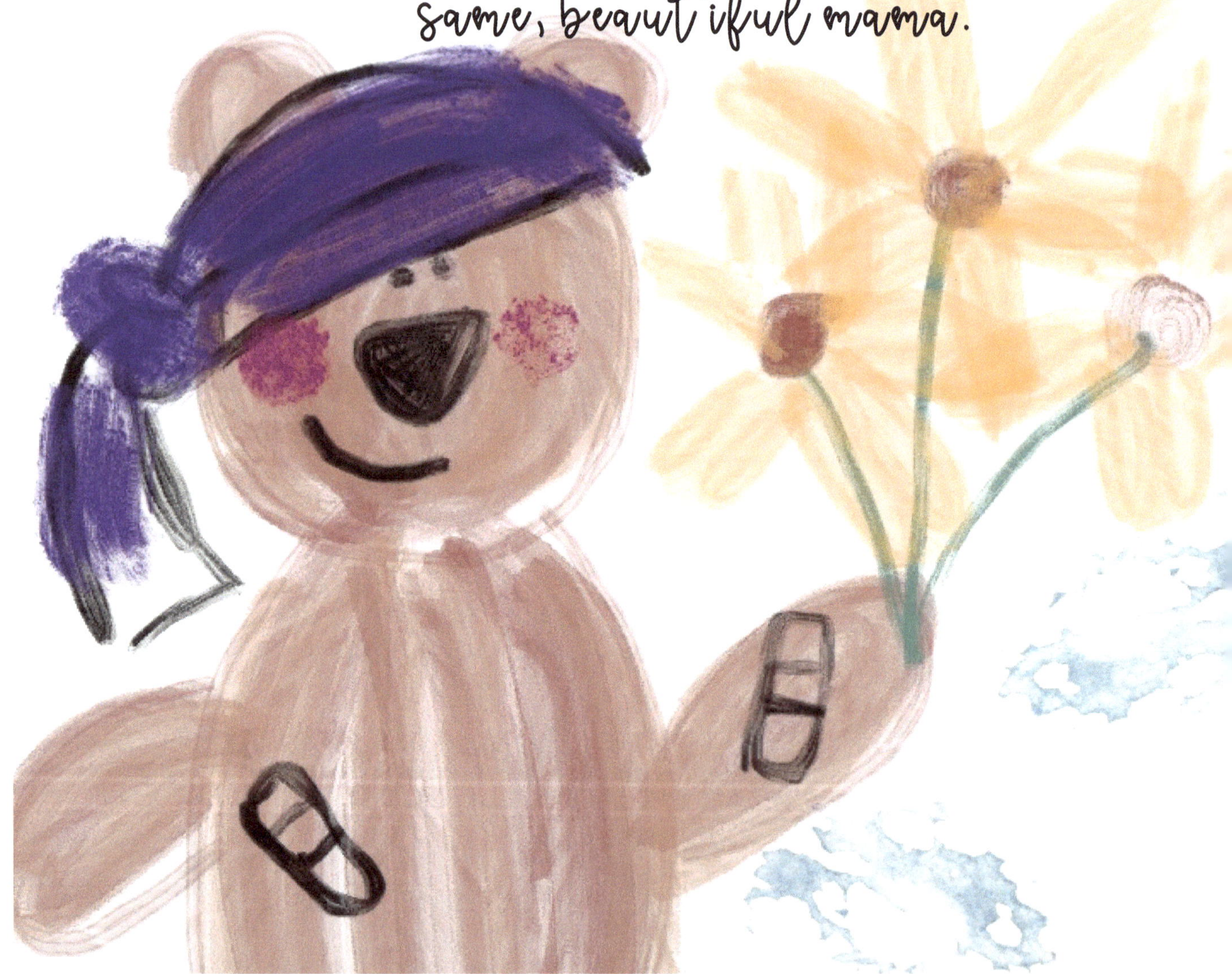

Even though some things are different a lot of my life is still the same.

I still have my pet fish (his name is pancake by the way).
I still love playing soccer, and
I still love playing with my friends everyday at school.

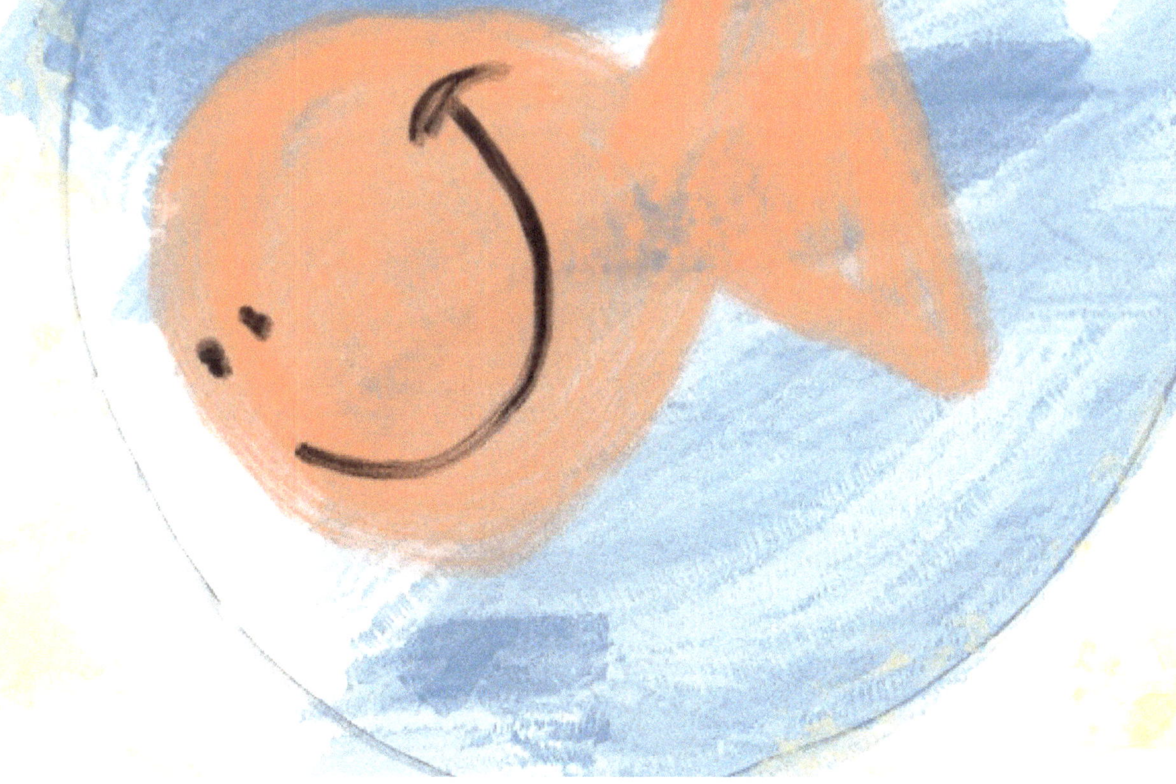

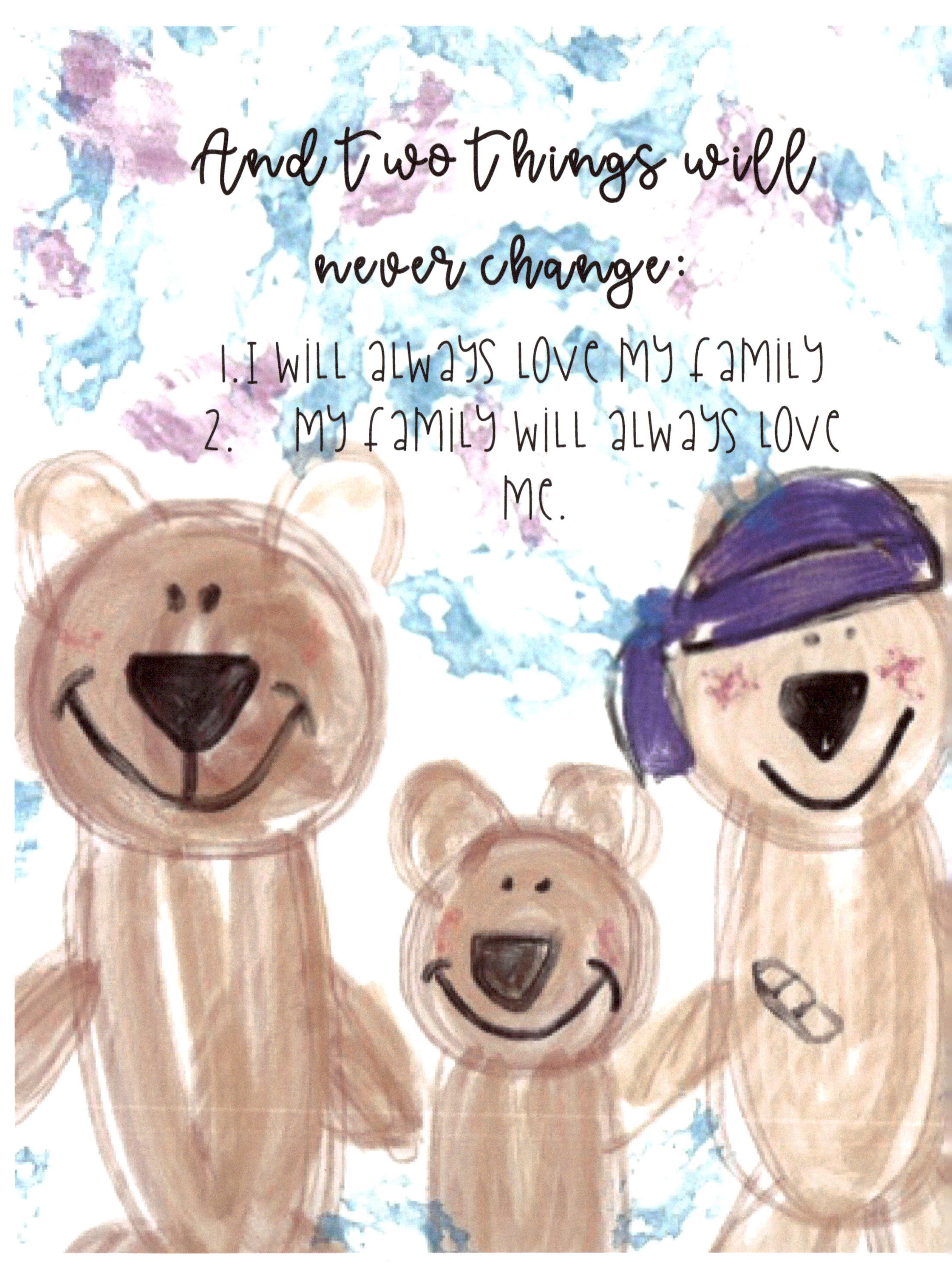

And two things will never change:
1. I will always love my family
2. My family will always love me.

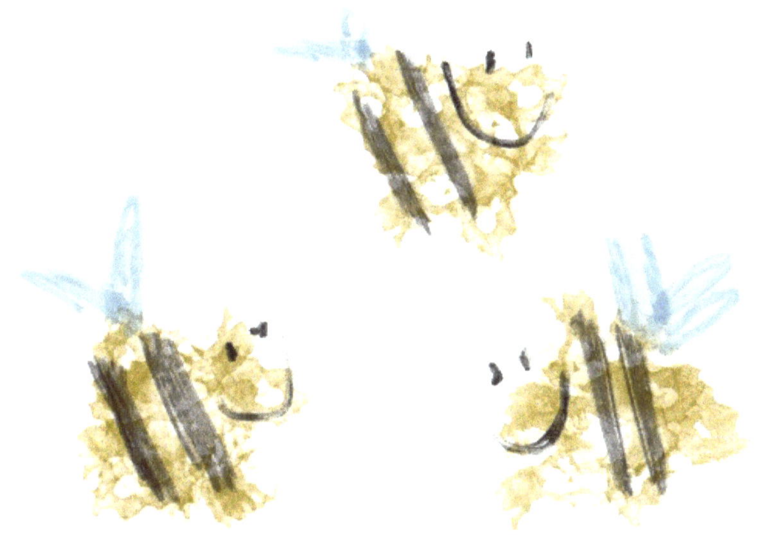

The end

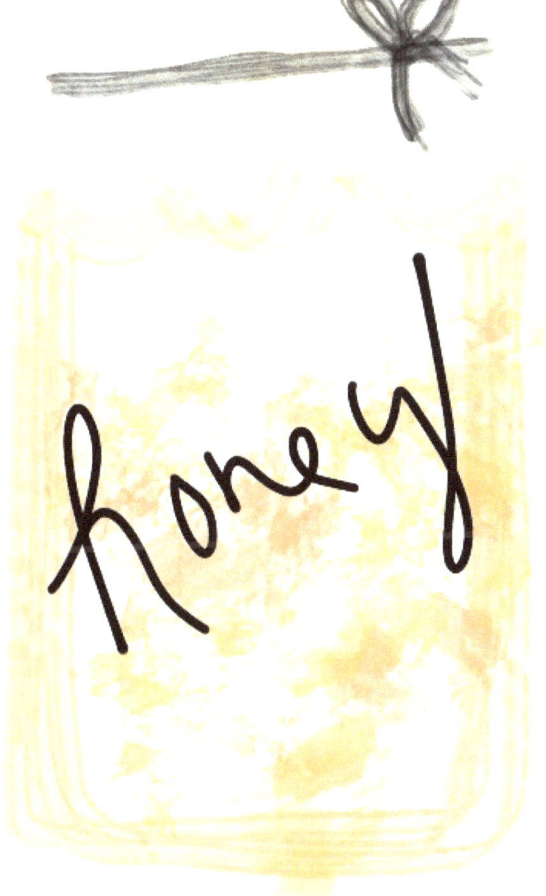

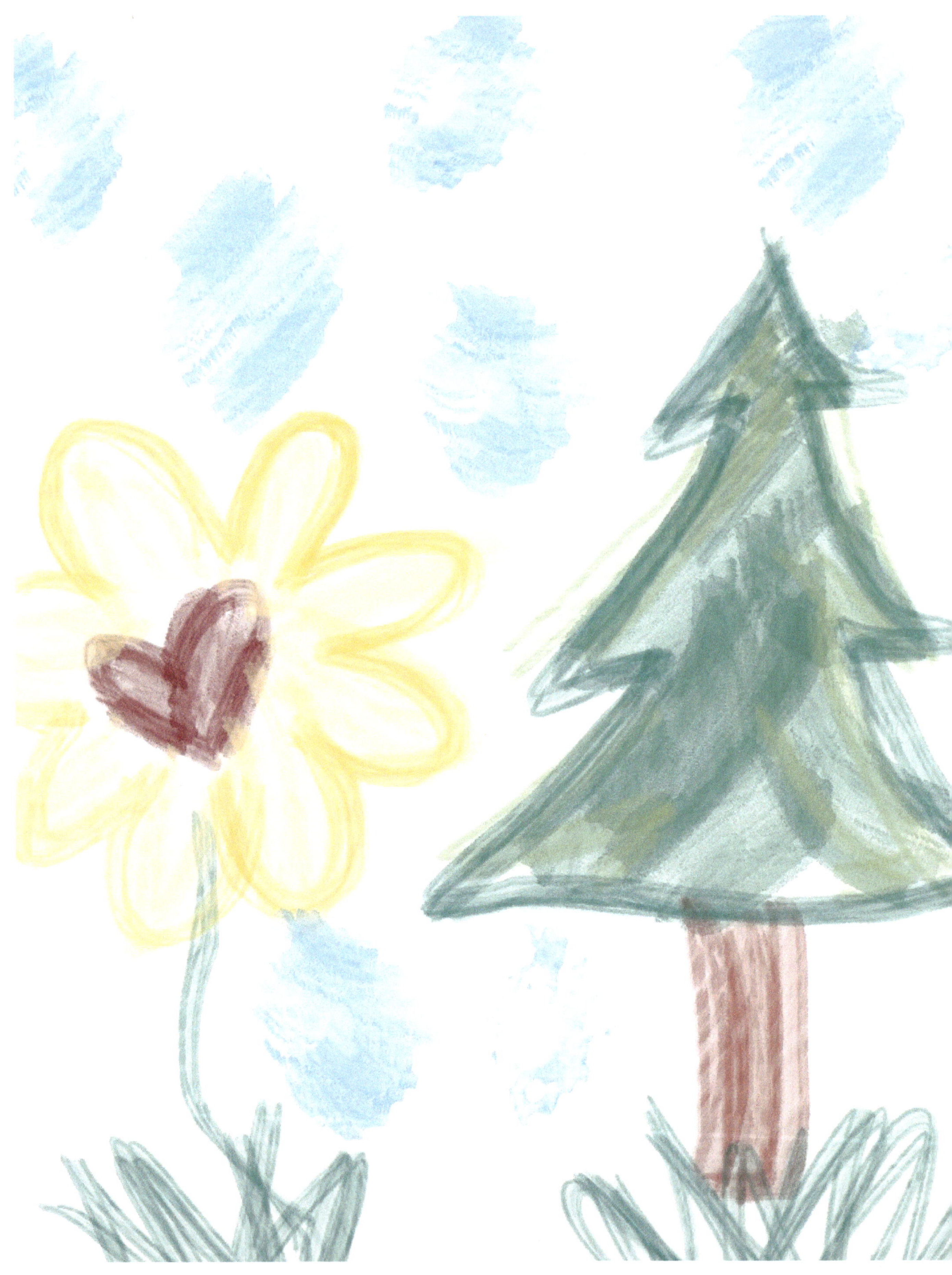